Table of Contents

Introduction

Crohn's disease is a chronic inflammatory bowel disease that can affect any part of the digestive tract, from the mouth to the anus. It is a debilitating condition that affects millions of people worldwide, and its cause is not yet fully understood. The disease causes inflammation, ulcers, and other complications that can interfere with normal digestion and nutrient absorption.

Crohn's disease is often characterized by symptoms such as abdominal pain, diarrhea, fatigue, and weight loss. The severity of these symptoms can vary from person to person and can change over time. While there is no cure for Crohn's disease, there are treatments available that can help manage symptoms and improve quality of life

Causes of Crohn's Disease

Crohn's disease is a chronic inflammatory bowel disease that affects the gastrointestinal tract. It can cause a range of symptoms, including abdominal pain, diarrhea, weight loss, and fatigue. The exact cause of Crohn's disease is unknown, but researchers believe that a combination of genetic and environmental factors may play a role.

Genetic factors are thought to contribute to the development of Crohn's disease. Studies have shown that people with a family history of the condition are at a higher risk of developing it themselves. There are several genes that have been associated with Crohn's disease, including NOD2, ATG16L1, and IRGM. These genes are involved in regulating the immune system and the response to bacteria in the gut.

Environmental factors may also play a role in the development of Crohn's disease. One theory is that the disease is caused by an abnormal immune response to bacteria in the gut. This could be triggered by a viral or bacterial infection, or exposure to certain environmental factors such as smoking, stress, or a diet high in processed foods and low in fiber.

Research has also suggested that the gut microbiome, which is the collection of microorganisms that live in the digestive tract, may play a role in the development of Crohn's disease. People with Crohn's disease have been found to have a less diverse microbiome, with a higher abundance of harmful bacteria and a lower abundance of beneficial bacteria. This imbalance in the microbiome could lead to inflammation and damage to the intestinal lining.

Symptoms of Crohn's Disease

Crohn's disease is a chronic inflammatory bowel disease that can affect any part of the gastrointestinal tract, from the mouth to the anus. It is characterized by inflammation and ulceration in the lining of the digestive tract, leading to various symptoms that can range from mild to severe.

The symptoms of Crohn's disease can vary greatly from person to person, depending on the location and severity of the inflammation. Common symptoms include:

Abdominal pain and cramping: This is often the first symptom of Crohn's disease. The pain can be constant or come and go, and may be accompanied by cramping or bloating.

Diarrhea: Chronic diarrhea is another hallmark symptom of Crohn's disease. The stools may be loose, watery, or contain mucus or blood.

Fatigue: Chronic inflammation and nutrient deficiencies can lead to fatigue and a general feeling of malaise.

Weight loss: The chronic inflammation and diarrhea associated with Crohn's disease can cause weight loss, especially if the disease is severe.

Anemia: Chronic inflammation and blood loss in the stool can lead to anemia, which can cause fatigue, weakness, and shortness of breath.

Nausea and vomiting: Inflammation in the upper part of the digestive tract can cause nausea and vomiting.

Joint pain: Crohn's disease is an autoimmune disorder, which means the body's immune system attacks its own tissues. This can lead to joint pain and inflammation.

Skin problems: Some people with Crohn's disease develop skin rashes or sores.

Eye problems: Inflammation in the eyes can cause redness, pain, and blurred vision.

Mouth sores: Inflammation in the mouth can cause painful sores.

It's important to note that not everyone with Crohn's disease will experience all of these symptoms, and some people may have very mild symptoms or no symptoms at all. In addition, the symptoms can come and go over time, with periods of remission alternating with flare-ups of the disease.

If you are experiencing any of these symptoms, it's important to talk to your doctor, who can perform diagnostic tests to determine if you have Crohn's disease or another condition. Early diagnosis and treatment are important for managing the symptoms of Crohn's disease and preventing complications

Other factors that may contribute to the development of Crohn's disease include a history of frequent antibiotic use, a weakened immune system, and certain medications, such as nonsteroidal anti-inflammatory drugs (NSAIDs) and oral contraceptives

Diagnosis of Crohn's Disease

Crohn's disease is a complex condition that can be challenging to diagnose. There is no single test that can definitively diagnose Crohn's disease, and healthcare providers rely on a combination of patient history, physical examination, laboratory tests, imaging studies, and endoscopy to make a diagnosis.

To diagnose Crohn's disease, healthcare providers typically start by taking a detailed medical history and conducting a physical examination. They will ask about symptoms such as abdominal pain, diarrhea, weight loss, and fatigue, as well as any family history of inflammatory bowel disease.

Laboratory tests may also be ordered to help diagnose Crohn's disease. These tests can include blood tests to check for inflammation and anemia, stool tests to look for signs of infection or inflammation, and genetic tests to look for specific markers associated with Crohn's disease.

Imaging studies, such as CT scans, MRIs, and ultrasounds, can also be helpful in diagnosing Crohn's disease. These tests can provide detailed images of the gastrointestinal tract and can help healthcare providers identify areas of inflammation or damage.

Finally, endoscopy is often used to diagnose Crohn's disease. During an endoscopy, a thin, flexible tube with a camera on the end is inserted into the digestive tract. This allows healthcare providers to visualize the lining of the digestive tract and take biopsies of any areas that appear abnormal.

It is important to note that the diagnosis of Crohn's disease can be a lengthy and complex process, and it may take several tests and appointments with healthcare providers to arrive at a definitive diagnosis. However, once a diagnosis is made, treatment can begin to help manage symptoms and improve quality of life

Nutritional Challenges of Crohn's Disease

Crohn's disease is a chronic inflammatory condition of the gastrointestinal tract that affects the ability of the body to digest and absorb nutrients. This means that individuals with Crohn's disease often face several nutritional challenges that can lead to malnutrition and other health problems. The following are some of the common nutritional challenges associated with Crohn's disease:

Malabsorption: The inflammation in the digestive tract caused by Crohn's disease can affect the body's ability to absorb nutrients from food. This can lead to malabsorption of nutrients such as fats, proteins, carbohydrates, vitamins, and minerals.

Loss of appetite: Individuals with Crohn's disease often experience a loss of appetite, which can make it difficult to consume enough nutrients to meet their body's needs.

Diarrhea: Diarrhea is a common symptom of Crohn's disease and can result in the loss of water, electrolytes, and nutrients such as potassium and magnesium.

Food intolerances: Crohn's disease can cause food intolerances, which means that certain foods can trigger symptoms such as abdominal pain, bloating, and diarrhea.

Reduced nutrient absorption due to medication: Some medications used to treat Crohn's disease can reduce the body's ability to absorb nutrients.

Increased nutrient needs: Individuals with Crohn's disease may have increased nutrient needs due to the inflammation in the body and the energy required to heal damaged tissues.

Fatigue: Chronic fatigue is a common symptom of Crohn's disease, which can affect the ability of individuals to prepare and consume nutritious meals.

To overcome these nutritional challenges, individuals with Crohn's disease may need to make dietary and lifestyle changes. This may include:

Working with a registered dietitian: A registered dietitian can help individuals with Crohn's disease develop a personalized nutrition plan that meets their specific nutrient needs and food intolerances.

Eating smaller, more frequent meals: Eating smaller, more frequent meals throughout the day can help individuals with Crohn's disease consume enough nutrients and manage symptoms such as diarrhea and abdominal pain.

Consuming nutrient-dense foods: Nutrient-dense foods such as lean proteins, whole grains, fruits, and vegetables can help individuals with Crohn's disease meet their nutrient needs and support their overall health.

Avoiding trigger foods: Avoiding trigger foods that can exacerbate symptoms such as abdominal pain, bloating, and diarrhea can help individuals with Crohn's disease manage their condition.

Taking supplements: Individuals with Crohn's disease may need to take supplements such as iron, vitamin B12, and vitamin D to meet their nutrient needs.

Managing stress: Stress can exacerbate symptoms of Crohn's disease, so managing stress through techniques such as meditation, yoga, and deep breathing can be helpful.

Staying hydrated: Drinking plenty of water and electrolyte-rich fluids can help individuals with Crohn's disease stay hydrated and replace fluids lost due to diarrhea.

team to develop a comprehensive treatment plan that includes medication, lifestyle changes, and dietary modifications.

Overall, eating a healthy diet and working with a healthcare team can help individuals with Crohn's disease manage their symptoms, improve their quality of life, and promote overall health and wellness.

Nutritious and Delicious Recipes for Managing Crohn's Disease Symptoms

Green Vegetables Soup

Ingredients

0.5 lbs or 240g broccoli

0.3 lbs or 150g mushrooms

2 leeks

2 celery stalks

30g of fresh parsley

2 tsp sea salt

1/2 tsp black pepper

34fl oz or 1l of water

1 tbsp olive oil

Directions

Chop the vegetables into medium-sized pieces.

Heat the olive oil in a deep pan and fry the leeks on medium heat until translucent.

Add the celery, mushrooms, broccoli, salt, and pepper. Cook for a further 5 minutes while stirring regularly.

Add 1 or 1.5 liters of water, depending on how thick or thin you like soups. Then, add the parsley.

Put the heat on high and bring it to a boil. Cover with a lid and let it simmer for 10 minutes.

Turn the heat off and let it cool down for a few minutes.

Blend using either a hand blender or a food processor, and the soup is ready to be enjoyed!

Creamy Beetroot Salad

Ingredients

1.4lbs or 650g of cooked beetroot

3 tbsp mayonnaise or olive oil

3 tbsp apple cider vinegar

2 tsp garlic powder

1 tsp sea salt

1/2 tsp black pepper

Directions

Chop the cooked (but unseasoned) beetroot in cubes and place them in a salad bowl.

Add all the ingredients to the bowl.

Mix until well combined.

It's ready! To garnish, add fresh dill or chopped chives.

Saffron Tea

Ingredients

6 rose buds

6 cardamom pods

1 cinnamon stick

1 pinch of saffron pistils

34fl oz or 1l of water

Directions

Bring the water to a boil.

Place all the ingredients in a teapot.

Add the freshly boiled water.

Let it steep for 7-10 minutes. It's ready, enjoy!

Honey Blackened Salmon

Ingredients

For the Blackened Salmon

4 (4-6 oz.) salmon filets

1 teaspoon smoked paprika

1/2 teaspoon garlic powder

1/2 teaspoon salt

1/4 teaspoon onion powder

1/4 teaspoon oregano

1/4 teaspoon parsley

1/4 teaspoon black pepper

1/8 teaspoon cayenne pepper

For the Honey Butter

3 tablespoons unsalted butter, softened

2 teaspoons honey

Instructions

To a small bowl, add smoked paprika, garlic powder, salt, onion powder, oregano, parsley, black pepper, and cayenne pepper. Mix together and set aside.

To a small bowl, add softened butter and honey. Using a spoon, mix together. Set aside.

Heat grill to medium high heat, around 350-400°F.

Pat salmon dry with a paper towel.

Season the flesh side of the salmon with blackening seasoning. Gently rub in so the seasoning sticks.

Place salmon on the grill skin side first. Grill for 6-8 minutes until the salmon releases.

Gently, flip the salmon and grill flesh side for 1-2 minutes until slight grill marks appear.

Remove salmon from the grill when internal temperature reaches 145°F.

Immediately place a dollop of butter on each salmon filet.

Garnish with parsley and lemon wedge. Serve.

Air Fryer Instructions:

Heat air fryer to 400°F.

Do steps 1- 5. Spray air fryer basket with cooking spray.

Place salmon skin side down in the the air fryer basket and cook for 9 minutes.

Remove and top with honey butter.

Optional: garnish with parsley and lemon wedge.

Potato Salad

Ingredients

1kg of new potatoes

4 tablespoons of olive oil (If you're on the low FODMAP diet, garlic-infused olive oil works great)

1/2 lime

5 tablespoons of plain dairy-free yoghurt (make sure you use PLAIN and not sweetened)

A handful of chopped fresh chives (also a great low FODMAP flavoring)

1 large apple, peeled and chopped

2 tablespoons of apple cider vinegar

1 tablespoon of dairy-free butter

Optional extras: Sauerkraut or grated carrot

Directions

Add your potatoes to a pan of cold water and cook for approx 15 minutes (keep checking on them as you don't want them to go too soft and end up with mashed potato!)

Meanwhile, chop your apple and, if using, grate your carrot.

In a small mixing bowl, start to make your dressing. First, add the olive oil and apple cider vinegar and mix.

Now stir in the dairy-free yogurt to the dressing.

Squeeze 1/2 a lime into the dressing and mix it all together. Now you've got your dressing!

Once potatoes are cooked (you can keep them on longer if you prefer a softer potato salad), drain and stir through 1 tablespoon of dairy-free butter.

.Add your potatoes to the large bowl with the apple and any other veggies your using.

Stir in your dressing and coat the potatoes as evenly as possible.

Add a sprinkle of chives to serve. You could also add in some sauerkraut if you have some.

Chicken and vegetable lasagne

spray oil

14oz lean chicken mince

1 onion, finely diced

1 red capsicum, finely diced

2 x 14oz cans chopped tomatoes

1 tablespoon dried Italian herbs

2 cups mashed cooked pumpkin

11oz frozen spinach, thawed, cooked, drained

13oz fresh lasagne sheets

14oz passata

½ cup grated edam cheese

Instructions

1Preheat oven to 360°F. Spray a non-stick frying pan with oil. Cook chicken mince for about 5 minutes until browned, breaking up lumps. Add onion, capsicum, tomatoes and herbs. Combine and heat through.

2Cut pasta sheets to fit lasagne dish. Layer chicken pasta sauce with pasta sheets then a layer of mashed pumpkin, then a layer of spinach. Continue this process and end with a layer of pasta.

3Pour passata over assembled lasagna and sprinkle cheese over top. Bake in oven for 30 minutes.Bottom of Form

Gluten-Free Fried Rice with Chicken

EQUIPMENT

1 non-stick pan

INGREDIENTS

2/3 cup Jasmine Rice uncooked

4 large Eggs whisked

1/4 cup Water

6 Cremini Mushrooms sliced

2 cups Snap Peas chopped

8 ounces Cooked Chicken Breast chopped

1/2 tsp Sea Salt divided

1/4 cup Chives plus more for garnish

INSTRUCTIONS

Cook the rice according to the directions on the package.

Heat a non-stick pan over medium heat. Add the eggs to the pan and move them around with a spatula continuously until fluffy, about two minutes. Transfer to a bowl.

In the same pan, heat the water over medium to medium-high heat. Add the mushrooms, snap peas, chicken and half the salt, scraping up any bits at the bottom of the pan. Cook for about five minutes, or until the water has absorbed and the mushrooms are soft, and the snap peas are tender crisp.

Stir in the scrambled eggs, cooked rice, and chives, breaking up any large chunks. Season with the remaining salt to taste. Divide into bowls and garnish with additional chives(optional). Enjoy!

Garden Frittata

Ingredients for a garden frittata:

4 large organic eggs

1/2 tsp. salt

1 medium tomato, chopped

1/2 green bell pepper

1 Tbsp. fresh chives, finely chopped (or 1 tsp. dried chives)

1/2 cup soft goat cheese (optional)

Directions to make a garden frittata:

Preheat oven to 400F. Spray large skillet with cooking spray and set aside.

In a large bowl, whisk eggs and salt, then add the chopped vegetables, chives, and goat cheese. Whisk to combine.

Pour mixture into skillet and sprinkle remaining goat cheese on top.

Bake for 15 minutes. Remove from oven and allow it to cool for 5 minutes before serving.

Mashed Potatoes

ingredients

1 lb yellow potatoes

1 1/2 tsp sea salt

4 TBSP chicken stock (or homemade bone broth)

1 TBSP dairy free milk

1/2 tsp garlic powder

Optional: chopped chives or scallions

instructions

Bring a large pot of water to a boil and wash, peel, and cut the potatoes into chunks.

Add the potatoes to the boiling water.

While the potatoes are cooking, chop the chives or scallions if using.

Once the potatoes can be pierced with a fork, drain the water but using the same pot, add the liquids a little at a time, mashing and combining as you go. Add the seasonings and more sea salt, if desired.

Add the mashed potatoes to a bowl and garnish or mix in the chives/scallions if using.

Top of Form

Bottom of Form

Prawn Bisque

Ingredients

1 pound large shrimp, peeled and deveined, shells reserved

4 cups seafood stock

3 tablespoons good olive oil

2 cups chopped baby marrow

1 stem of celery

1 tablespoon chopped garlic

Pinch cayenne pepper

1/4 cup Cognac or brandy

1/4 cup dry sherry

4 tablespoons (1/2 stick) unsalted butter

1/4 cup all-purpose flour

2 cups half-and-half

1/3 cup roasted butternut squash and a bit of carrot juice

2 teaspoons kosher salt

1 teaspoon freshly ground black pepper

Instructions

Place the shrimp shells and seafood stock in a saucepan and simmer for 15 minutes.

Strain and reserve the stock. Add enough water to make 3 3/4 cups.

Meanwhile, heat the olive oil in a large pot or Dutch oven.

Add the leeks and cook them for 10 minutes over medium-low heat, or until the leeks are tender but not browned.

Add the garlic and cook for 1 more minute.

Add the cayenne pepper and shrimp and cook over medium to low heat for 3 minutes, stirring occasionally.

Add the Cognac and cook for 1 minute, then the sherry and cook for 3 minutes longer.

Transfer the shrimp and leeks to a food processor fitted with a steel blade and process until coarsely pureed.

In the same pot, melt the butter.

Add the flour and cook over medium-low heat for 1 minute, stirring with a wooden spoon.

Add the half-and-half and cook, stirring with a whisk, until thickened, about 3 minutes.

Stir in the pureed shrimp, the stock, tomato paste, salt, and pepper, and heat gently until hot but not boiling.

Season, taste, and serve hot.

Bolognese Sauce

Ingredients

600g or 21oz of lean beef minced

1 can of chopped tomatoes (400ml or 14oz)

4 garlic cloves

1 medium onion (or 2 small)

1 medium carrot (or 2 small)

1 tsp of sea salt

½ tsp of ground pepper

1 tsp of cinnamon

1 bsp of olive oil

Fresh basil to decorate

Directions

Finely chop the carrot and onion.

Heat the olive oil on medium in a large pan and add the crushed garlic, finely chopped onion, and carrot

Cook for about 5 minutes until the onion becomes translucent.

Add the minced meat and brown it

Add the tomatoes, salt, pepper, cinnamon and bring to a simmer.

Cook on low to medium for about 40 minutes, until the sauce is reduced.

Taste and add salt if needed. Make sure to stir regularly.

Once cooked, serve on zucchini noodles or on a bed of steamed broccolini and decorate with finely chopped basil leaves

Maple Syrup

EQUIPMENT

1 Saucepan

1 Stove

INGREDIENTS

1x2x3x

1 Cup Water

1 Cup Maple Syrup

3 Cups Cranberries Fresh or frozen

INSTRUCTIONS

Combine water and maple syrup in a saucepan and bring to a boil.

Add cranberries and cook until they burst and soften, about 20 to 25 minutes. Let cool before serving. Enjoy!

NOTES

Serving SizeOne serving is equal to approximately 1/4 cup of cranberry sauce.

LeftoversRefrigerate in an airtight container up to one week or freeze for up to three months.

Serve it WithTurkey, stuffing, brie, as a jam, with yogurt or in baked goods.

Blueberry Ginger Lime Sparkling Water

EQUIPMENT

Mason jars or glasses

INGREDIENTS

1/2 cup blueberries

1 lime sliced

1 Tbsp ginger peeled and sliced

6 ice cubes

3 cups sparkling water

INSTRUCTIONS

Divide blueberries, lime slices, ginger, and ice between mason jars or glasses.

Top with sparkling water.

Enjoy!

Chocolate & Strawberry Yogurt Bark

EQUIPMENT

1 Baking Sheet

1 Large Bowl

1 Mixing Spoon

parchment paper

Freezer

INGREDIENTS

2 cups Plain Greek Yogurt

1 Tbsp Maple Syrup

1/2 tsp Vanilla Extract

1/2 cup Strawberries

1 cup Granola

3/4 oz Dark Chocolate chopped

INSTRUCTIONS

Line a baking sheet with parchment paper.

Stir the yogurt, maple syrup, and vanilla extract together in a bowl. Pour the mixture onto the baking sheet and evenly spread it out.

Top with granola, strawberries, and dark chocolate.Set in the freezer overnight. Break apart and enjoy

Avocado Pudding

EQUIPMENT

food processor or high-speed blender

INGREDIENTS

2 large avocados

4 tsp vanilla extract

2 medium bananas preferably ripe with spots

2 Tbsp honey

INSTRUCTIONS

Blend ingredients together.

Buffalo Chicken Mac & Cheese

ingredients

1 lb gluten free pasta or a veggie pasta (i.e. zoodles)

4 tbsp grass-fed butter

3 tbsp tapioca flour

2 cups coconut milk

4 oz grass-fed cream cheese (1/2 a block)

1 1/2 cups Monterey Jack cheese

1 cup shredded mozzarella

2 tsp sea salt

1 1/2 tsp garlic powder

2 cups shredded chicken

1 cup hot sauce

Optional: dried or fresh herbs for garnish or extra hot sauce

instructions

Boil the pasta as you normally would in a large pot. Drain once done and set aside. Turn the heat down to medium.

In the same pot, add the butter and whisk while sprinkling in the tapioca flour. Slowly pour in the coconut milk while continuing to whisk.

Add in the cream cheese, Monterey Jack, and mozzarella cheeses. Stir continuously until everything has melted together and there are no lumps.

Add the sea salt and garlic powder.

In bowl with the shredded chicken, add the hot sauce. Stir to coat then add to the pot. Add the pasta back to the pot as well. Stir until everything is well incorporated and transfer to a bowl to serve.

If you desire, add a drizzle of hot sauce on top and/or dried or fresh herbs like parsley, basil, or chives.

Blueberry Lemon Cookies

INGREDIENTS

2 1/4 cups AP flour can be substituted for gluten free flour

3/4 tsp baking soda

1/4 tsp salt

1/3 cup coconut sugar

1/3 cup honey

1 large egg

1 tsp vanilla

6 Tbsp coconut oil melted

1/4 cup lemon juice

1 cup frozen blueberries

1/8 cup extra frozen blueberries

1/2 cup powdered sugar

1 Tbsp non-dairy milk such as oat milk, almond milk, cashew milk, or soy milk

1 tsp lemon zest

INSTRUCTIONS

Preheat oven to 350°F.

Finely zest two lemons using a microplane.

In a large bowl, mix together flour, baking soda, and salt.

In a separate large bowl, add 1 cup of frozen blueberries.

Either in the microwave or on the stovetop, thaw the frozen blueberries until they're soft and jammy. (In the microwave this should take about 30 seconds over high heat, and on the stovetop it should take about 2-3 minutes on medium heat.)

Let the blueberries cool for about 2-3 minutes.

Add coconut sugar, honey, egg, vanilla, coconut oil, and lemon juice to the thawed blueberry mixture.

Mix at a high speed. You want to "mash" the blueberries into the mixture, making it so that they are puréed and fully combined with the other ingredients. The mixture should be a deep purple color.

Add dry ingredients to wet ingredients and mix until well combined.

Line a large baking sheet with parchment paper.

Scoop out 2-Tablespoons worth of batter and place onto the baking sheet. Repeat with remaining cookie dough, making sure they are all at least 2-inches apart.

Place 2-3 additional blueberries on the surface of the cookie dough balls.

Bake cookies in a preheated oven for 13-15 minutes, or until the edges are slightly golden.

While the cookies are baking, whisk together the lemon glaze ingredients in a small bowl (powdered sugar, non-dairy milk, and lemon zest).

Once cookies have cooled to room temperature, drizzle lemon glaze over each one.

Egg White Cups with Veggies

EQUIPMENT

Sauté Pan

Bowl

Muffin pan

Parchment paper muffin cups

INGREDIENTS

1 Tbsp olive oil

2 cups fresh spinach

2 stalks green onion chopped

8 mushrooms sliced

1 1/2 tsp Italian Seasoning

8 egg whites

1/4 cup Parmesan cheese grated or shredded (Optional, but used in nutrition analysis)

6 cherry tomatoes sliced in quarters

INSTRUCTIONS

In a pan, add olive oil and sauté green onions and mushrooms on medium-low heat for about 3-5 minutes. Add Italian Seasoning and mix into sautéed mushrooms and onions. Then add spinach and cook for an additional 2 minutes on low-heat. Place sautéed vegetable aside.

Separate eggs using only the egg whites. In a bowl, whip egg whites with a fork until there are foamy bubbles.

Place parchment paper muffin cups into muffin baking pan. Pour about 1/4 cup egg white into muffin pan, about halfway full. Scoop one spoonful of sautéed veggies into each cup (use a teaspoon). Optional: sprinkle Parmesan cheese on top of each mini quiche followed by a couple of tomato slices.

Bake at 350°F for about 20-30 minutes. Quiche tops should become golden brown. Remove from oven. Let cool 5 minutes and remove parchment paper. Place on serving dish and serve!

Chocolate Chip Cookies

INGREDIENTS

1x2x3x

1/2 cup coconut oil

1 1/4 cups brown sugar packed

2 tsp vanilla extract

1/4 cup oat milk or plant-based milk of choice

1/4 cup unsweetened applesauce

1 1/3 cup enriched all-purpose flour sifted

1 tsp salt

1 1/2 cups chocolate chips type and brand of choice

INSTRUCTIONS

Preheat oven to 375°F.

Line a large baking sheet with parchment paper; set aside.

In a large bowl, whisk together the coconut oil, brown sugar, and vanilla, beating until well combined.

Add in the oat milk and applesauce and whisk until well combined; set aside.

In a separate bowl, combine the flour, baking soda, and salt. Whisk well to combine.

Add the dry ingredients into the wet mixture. Stir ingredients until combined using a wooden spoon or very study spatula.

Fold in chocolate chips.

Scoop cookie dough onto the prepared cooking sheet, leaving at least an inch in between cookies for spreading.

Bake for 9-10 minutes, or until the cookie edges are golden and the centers have set.

Cool cookies on the baking sheet for 15 minutes before transferring them to a cooling rack.

Spiced Pancakes with Orange Zest

INGREDIENTS

Pancake Ingredients

2 3/4 cups all-purpose flour add more if batter is thin

1 1/2 tsp baking powder

1/2 tsp baking soda

1/2 tsp salt

1 1/2 tsp Pumpkin Pie Spice

2 3/4 cups oat, almond, or hazelnut milk oat milk was used in the nutritional analysis

2 large eggs

2 Tbsp coconut oil or butter melted

1/4 cup sugar

1 medium orange, skin zested Use half for batter. Save other half for topping of pancakes

non-stick cooking spray or butter for pan

Optional Topping Ingredients

maple syrup

3 Tbsp powdered sugar

1 Tbsp Pumpkin Pie Spice

sprinkle granola

INSTRUCTIONS

Pancake Instructions

In a large bowl, combine flour, baking powder, baking soda, salt and pumpkin pie spice. Mix well.

In a medium size bowl mix milk, eggs, butter, sugar. Beat with whisk. Mix well.

Combine wet ingredients with dry ingredients. Using a whisk, mix, but do not over-mix! There will be lumps in the batter — this is normal!

Let batter sit for 5 minutes.

Heat up pan. Once pan is hot spray with cooking spray or melt butter into pan. Pour batter into pan.

Flip pancakes once bubbles form on the top of the pancakes and check underside for a nice golden-brown color.

Cook second side until golden brown and remove onto serving plate.

Potential Topping Instructions

Combine powdered sugar and pumpkin pie spice. Mix well. Place pancakes onto plate, drizzle syrup, then powdered sugar with cinnamon. Sprinkle some orange zest. For people who like a crunch, add granola.

Spiced Banana Almond Milk Smoothie

EQUIPMENT

Blender

INGREDIENTS

4 cups unsweetened almond milk preferably with only almonds & water

1 medium banana preferably with spots

2 Tbsp honey

1 tsp Pumpkin Pie Spice

INSTRUCTIONS

Place all ingredients into a blender and mix well.

Cucumber Tuna Bites

EQUIPMENT

Small bowl

INGREDIENTS

1 can Tuna flaked and drained

1 large Cucumber peeled, sliced into rounds

2 Tbsp Mayonnaise

INSTRUCTIONS

Add the tuna and the mayonnaise to a small bowl and mix together.

Top each cucumber round with a spoonful of the tuna mixture.

Enjoy!

Peanut Butter Rice

EQUIPMENT

1 Loaf Pan greased

1 Medium Pot

1 Whisk

1 Spatula

INGREDIENTS

1 TBSP Coconut Oil

1/2 Cup Maple Syrup

1/2 Cup Peanut Butter All-Natural

2 1/2 Cups Rice Puffs Cereal

INSTRUCTIONS

Grease a loaf pan with coconut oil or line with parchment paper (use a larger baking dish if serving size is adjusted higher).

In a medium pot over low-medium heat, whisk together maple syrup and peanut butter until thoroughly combined. Remove from heat and let cool, about 5 minutes.

Add puffed rice and gently mix with a spatula until evenly coated

Transfer to loaf pan and press down firmly. Freeze for 20 minutes or until firm. Slice into bars or squares and enjoy!

Mango Nice Cream

INGREDIENTS

4 cups frozen mango

2 cups oat milk or your favorite non-dairy milk like: coconut, cashew, or almond milk.

INSTRUCTIONS

Blend mango and oat milk in a blender or food processor until smooth.

Transfer mango puree into popsicle molds, individual paper containers, a baking pan, or insulated tub.

Freeze for 4-6 hours.

Serve and enjoy!

Salmon & Veggie Skewers with Herbed Yogurt Dip

EQUIPMENT

Metal or bamboo skewers

INGREDIENTS

4 Tbsp avocado oil

3 Tbsp Italian Seasoning divided; see notes section for more info

1 1/2 lbs salmon without skin, cut into 1 inch cubes

12 whole mushrooms

12 cherry tomatoes

1 cup plain non-fat Greek yogurt or unsweetened coconut yogurt (plain nonfat Greek yogurt used in nutritional analysis)

1/2 cucumber grated

INSTRUCTIONS

Salmon Skewer Instructions

Using a small bowl, add 3 Tbsp. avocado oil and 1 Tbsp. Italian Seasoning and mix well.

Place your one inch salmon into a bowl. Place your cut up vegetable into a separate bowl.

Using a spoon drizzle flavored avocado oil over vegetables and mix well so all veggies are coated with avocado oil. Repeat with salmon and mix well so all pieces of fish are well coated.

Using skewers, place fish and vegetables onto skewers alternating fish and veggies until everything is used up.

Pre-heat grill to 500°F. Reduce heat to about 400°F.

Place skewers on grill. Cook until there is are nice grill marks and then turn skewers so all sides are cooked evenly. Remove when fish has reached an internal temperature of 140°F.

Let rest for a couple of minutes.

Yogurt Dip Instructions

Place yogurt into a medium size bowl with 2 Tbsp. Italian Seasoning, 1 cup yogurt, and grated cucumber. Mix well and serve with salmon & veggie skewers.

Almond Milk Rice Pudding

EQUIPMENT

1 Pot Large

1 Mixing Spoon Large

3 Bowls or Jars For storage

1 Fridge and/or Freezer

INGREDIENTS

3 cups unsweetened almond milk

1/4 cup maple syrup

2 tsps vanilla extract

1/8 tsp sea salt

1/2 cup arborio rice

1/8 tsp cinnamon ground

INSTRUCTIONS

In a large pot combine the almond milk, maple syrup, vanilla and sea salt and stir together. Over medium heat, bring the almond milk mixture to a gentle boil. Stir in the rice and reduce heat to low.

Allow the rice to gently simmer and stir often. Every 3 to 5 minutes is best to prevent sticking and to help the pudding thicken. Continue for 20 to 25 minutes or until the rice is tender, the liquid has absorbed and the pudding has thickened.

Remove from the heat and let the rice pudding cool in the pot for 10 minutes. It will continue to thicken as it cools. Divide the warm pudding evenly between bowls. Sprinkle with cinnamon and enjoy!

Pan Seared Salmon with Sage Brown Butter Sauce

Ingredients

2 tablespoons olive oil

6 (4 oz) salmon filets, skin on

1 teaspoon sea salt

6 tablespoons unsalted butter

1 1/2 teaspoons raw honey

1 teaspoon diced fresh sage

1/4 teaspoon ground nutmeg

1/4 teaspoon sea salt

Instructions

Bring a large skillet to medium high heat.

Pat the salmon dry and season the flesh side of the salmon using 1 teaspoon of sea salt.

Add the olive oil to the hot skillet and immediately add the salmon to the pan flesh side down. Saute the salmon for 4-5 minutes until browned.

Gently flip the salmon to saute on the skin side for another 4-6 minutes. (it may take longer depending on thickness of your salmon. Remove from pan and let sit to cool.

In the meantime, bring a small skillet to medium heat.

Add butter and 1/4 teaspoon of sea salt to the pan and melt.

Once the butter is melted, add the honey, sage, and nutmeg. Stir and let the butter begin to brown, for about 5 minutes. Be sure to stir throughout cooking process so the butter does not burn. Remove from heat.

Serve salmon with drizzle of sage brown butter sauce. (i used about 1 tablespoon for each salmon filet)

Avocado Pudding

EQUIPMENT

food processor or high-speed blender

INGREDIENTS

2 large avocados

4 tsp vanilla extract

2 medium bananas preferably ripe with spots

2 Tbsp honey

INSTRUCTIONS

Blend ingredients together.

Banana Pancakes

INGREDIENTS

1 cup all purpose flour

1 Tbsp coconut sugar

2 tsp baking powder

1/4 tsp salt

1 large egg, beaten

1 cup non-dairy milk

2 Tbsp high-heat oil

2 ripe bananas, mashed

1/2 tsp vanilla extract optional

INSTRUCTIONS

Combine flour, sugar, baking powder, and salt in a medium bowl.

In a separate large bowl, mix together egg, milk, oil, and bananas.

Stir flour mixture into banana mixture (batter will be slightly lumpy)

Heat a lightly oiled griddle or pan over medium heat.

Pour or scoop the batter onto the griddle, using approximately 1/4 cup for each pancake.

Cook until pancakes are golden brown on both sides; serve right away.

Gingerbread Chocolate Chip Cookies

EQUIPMENT

oven

Large baking sheet

parchment paper

2 Large bowls

Handheld electric mixer

INGREDIENTS

1/2 cup coconut oil, solid be sure it's not melted at all

3/4 cup dark brown sugar, packed

1/2 cup granulated sugar

2 tsp vanilla extract

2 Tbsp unsulphured molasses

2 Tbsp non-dairy milk oat milk used in nutrition analysis

1/3 cup pumpkin puree not pumpkin pie mix

2 1/4 cups all-purpose flour, sifted (for GF replacement, please see above notes)

1 tsp baking soda

1 tsp salt

2 tsp Pumpkin Pie Spice

3/4 cup mini semi-sweet chocolate chips dairy-free (I used Enjoy Life brand)

INSTRUCTIONS

Preheat oven to 375°F. Line a large baking sheet with parchment paper; set aside.

In a large bowl using a handheld electric mixer, beat the coconut oil, both sugars, and vanilla on medium-speed until smooth; about 2 minutes.

Add in the molasses, oat milk, and pumpkin puree and beat on low speed until well combined.

In a separate bowl, combine the flour, baking soda, salt, and Pumpkin Pie Spice; whisk well to combine.

Add the dry ingredients into the wet mixture and, with the mixer on low speed, beat until ingredients are combined. The batter will be very thick! Fold in chocolate chips.

Scoop tablespoon-sized mounds of dough onto the prepared cookie sheet, leaving a few inches between each cookie. Bake for 9 to 10 minutes, or until the edges are golden and the centers are soft but set.

Cool cookies on the baking sheet for 30 minutes before transferring them to a cooling rack.

Poke Bowl with Spicy

Ingredients

For the Salmon Poke

1 lb. raw salmon skin removed, cut into 1" cubes

2 teaspoons toasted sesame oil

2 1/2 tablespoons tamari sauce

1/2 tablespoon rice wine vinegar

1 garlic clove, minced

1 teaspoon fresh ginger, minced

1 teaspoon black sesame seeds

For the Sriracha Mayo Sauce

3 tablespoons mayo

3 teaspoons sriracha

For the Bowls

2 bags of Success Basmati Boil-in-Bag Rice

2 cups cucumber, thinly sliced

1 cup edamame

1 avocado, thinly sliced

1 cup mango, diced

1 cup sliced scallions

Instructions

Make the Salmon Poke

To a large bowl add sesame oil, tamari sauce, rice wine vinegar, garlic, ginger and black sesame seeds. Whisk to combine.

Add cubes salmon to the bowl. Toss to coat the salmon with the sauce and let marinate for 10 minutes.

Preheat oven to 400°F.

Add salmon cubes to a tin foil lined baking sheet and bake for 8 minutes. Remove and let rest.

Boil the Rice

Add 8 cups of water to a pot. Submerge Success Bastami rice bag into the water. Bring to a boil and boil uncovered for 10 minutes. Remove bag immediately from water with a fork, drain, empty rice into serving dish and fluff with fork. Set aside.

Make the Sriracha

To a small bowl add mayonnaise and sriracha. Stir with a spoon until combined. Set aside.

Assemble the Bowls

To a bowl add 1 cup of basmati rice, 1/2 cup sliced cucumber, 1/4 cup edamame, 1/4 of an avocado, 1/4 cup of diced mango, 1/4 cup of scallions, 4 -6 oz. of cubes salmon and drizzle with sriracha mayo.

Serve!

Healthy Chocolate Chip Pumpkin Muffins

EQUIPMENT

1 Muffin Tray

12 Muffin liners

1 Bowl Large

1 oven

INGREDIENTS

1 tbsp Ground Flax Seed

3 tbsps Water

1 can Pureed Pumpkin

1/4 cup Oat Milk

1/3 cup Coconut Sugar

1/4 cup Coconut Oil

1 1/3 cups Oat Flour

1/2 cup Cocoa Powder

2 tsps Pumpkin Pie Spice

1 tsp Baking Powder

1/2 tsp Baking Soda

1/4 tsp Sea Salt

1/2 cup Dark Chocolate Chips (optional)

INSTRUCTIONS

Preheat the oven to 350ºF (177ºC) and line a muffin tray with liners or use a silicone muffin tray.

In a large bowl combine the ground flax and water. Let it sit for five minutes or until thickened.

To the same bowl, add the pumpkin, oat milk, coconut sugar, and coconut oil. Mix until smooth. Then add the oat flour, cocoa powder, pumpkin pie spice, baking powder, baking soda, and salt. Stir well until combined. Fold in the chocolate chips, if using.

Fill each muffin liner about 3/4 full and place in the oven to bake for 22 to 25 minutes, until cooked through. Remove from the oven and let cool before serving or storing. Enjoy!

CHICKEN TURMERIC RICE

Ingredients

3 tbsp olive oil OR garlic infused oil

4 chicken drumsticks skinless

1 tbsp turmeric

1 cup | 220 gr white rice medium-grain

1 large carrot finely chopped

1/2 cup chickpeas canned

sea salt

Instructions

Heat the olive oil in a large non-stick frying pan over medium–high heat.

Toss in the chicken and turmeric and cook for 2–3 minutes, or until golden brown, turning often to ensure even color.

Cover the chicken with water and let it cook over medium heat for approx. 20 minutes, stirring occasionally.

Add the rice, carrot, chickpeas and cover again with water. Bring to the boil, salt to taste, then reduce the heat to low. Cover and simmer for another 15 minutes until all the water is absorbed and the rice is tender. Give everything a good stir and season to taste, if necessary.

Remove from the heat and stand, covered, for a further 15 minutes.

HONEY GARLIC BUTTER SHRIMP & BROCCOLI

INGREDIENTS

1/2 cup honey

1/4 cup soy sauce

1 teaspoon fresh grated ginger

2 tablespoons minced garlic

1/4 teaspoon red pepper flakes

1/2 teaspoon cornstarch

1 pound large shrimp, peeled, deveined and tails removed if desired

2 tablespoon butter

2 cups chopped broccoli

1 teaspoon olive oil

salt pepper

INSTRUCTIONS

In a small bowl add the honey, soy sauce, ginger, garlic, red pepper, and mix until combined.

Place the peeled and deveined shrimp into a bowl and add 1/3 of the sauce. Toss and marinate for 30 minutes.

Whisk in the cornstarch to the reserved marinade and set aside.

Heat a skillet (I use cast iron) or wok on high heat, add olive oil and broccoli, salt and pepper and cook 5-6 minutes just until soft. Remove from pan and set aside.

Add the butter to the skillet and add shrimp discarding any marinade. Cook until the shrimp turns pink about 2 minutes on each side.

Add in the reserved sauce and bring to a simmer. Add in the broccoli and toss until heated through.

Serve with white rice or pasta.

Garnish with green onions if desired.

Conclusion

Cooking for Crohn's provides nutritious and delicious recipes for managing Crohn's disease symptoms. Crohn's disease is a chronic condition that affects the digestive system, leading to inflammation and discomfort. While there is no cure for Crohn's disease, following a healthy and balanced diet can help manage symptoms and improve overall health and well-being.

The recipes in this cookbook are designed to be easy to prepare, flavorful, and packed with nutrients that support digestive health. By following the guidelines and tips for eating with Crohn's disease, individuals can better manage their symptoms and maintain a healthy and satisfying diet.

Cooking for Crohn's aims to provide a comprehensive resource for individuals with Crohn's disease, their families, and caregivers. With the right knowledge and tools, individuals can take control of their health and lead a fulfilling life despite their condition.

This cookbook is not just about managing Crohn's disease symptoms but also about enjoying the pleasure of food.

The recipes are not only nutritious but also delicious, making it easy to maintain a healthy and satisfying diet. Cooking for Crohn's is a valuable resource for anyone looking to manage their Crohn's disease symptoms through nutrition and healthy eating.

www.ingramcontent.com/pod-product-compliance
Lightning Source LLC
Chambersburg PA
CBHW061601250726
48657CB00020B/905